LICHEN SCLEROSUS DIET

A Beginner's 3-Week Guide for Women, With
Curated Recipes and a Sample Meal Plan

Stephanie Hinderock

mindplusfood

Disclaimer

By reading this disclaimer, you are accepting the terms of the disclaimer in full. If you disagree with this disclaimer, please do not read the guide.

All of the content within this guide is provided for informational and educational purposes only, and should not be accepted as independent medical or other professional advice. The author is not a doctor, physician, nurse, mental health provider, or registered nutritionist/dietician. Therefore, using and reading this guide does not establish any form of a physician-patient relationship.

Always consult with a physician or another qualified health provider with any issues or questions you might have regarding any sort of medical condition. Do not ever disregard any qualified professional medical advice or delay seeking that advice because of anything you have read in this guide. The information in this guide is not intended to be any sort of medical advice and should not be used in lieu of any medical advice by a licensed and qualified medical professional.

The information in this guide has been compiled from a variety of known sources. However, the author cannot attest to or guarantee the accuracy of each source and thus should not be held liable for any errors or omissions.

You acknowledge that the publisher of this guide will not be held liable for any loss or damage of any kind incurred as a result of this guide or the reliance on any information provided within this guide. You acknowledge and agree that you assume all risk and responsibility for any action you undertake in response to the information in this guide.

Using this guide does not guarantee any particular result (e.g., weight loss or a cure). By reading this guide, you acknowledge that there are no guarantees to any specific outcome or results you can expect.

All product names, diet plans, or names used in this guide are for identification purposes only and are the property of their respective owners. The use of these names does not imply endorsement. All other trademarks cited herein are the property of their respective owners.

Where applicable, this guide is not intended to be a substitute for the original work of this diet plan and is, at most, a supplement to the original work for this diet plan and never a direct substitute. This guide is a personal expression of the facts of that diet plan.

Where applicable, persons shown in the cover images are stock photography models and the publisher has obtained the rights to use the images through license agreements with third-party stock image companies.

CONTENTS

INTRODUCTION

L ichen sclerosus or LS is a lingering, fiery skin illness. It causes white, thin, patchy parts of skin that may feel itchy and painful and may even tear and bleed. This usually affects the skin around the genitalia and anus but also affects other parts of the upper body, such as the breasts and the upper arms.

How the condition is acquired is still commonly unknown to doctors, but cases have been noted that it affects men and women, children and adults alike. According to a study. It is ten times more common in women than in men, prevalent in 1 out of 30 older women and 1 in 900 girls before they reach puberty. There is no cure to completely eradicate this condition, but there are several ways to make living with it bearable.

There are several treatments to alleviate the pain and discomfort caused by LS. Another way to support these treatments is to follow a diet program that will be beneficial to you, which is called the lichen sclerosus diet.

In this guide, you will discover the following:
• What lichen sclerosus is about
• How it affects people
• Symptoms and treatments
• What foods to eat and avoid when diagnosed with LS

Whether you're curious about this condition or are diagnosed with it and are trying to find alternative ways to deal with LS, this guide will be useful in providing that information.

UNDERSTANDING LICHEN SCLEROSUS

Lichen sclerosus, known in the scientific field as lichen sclerosus et atrophicus, or LS in simpler terms, is a persistent, inflammatory skin condition that usually affects the genital and anal areas. It shows up as white patches on the skin that may cause discomfort, itchiness, and tearing or bleeding. It is most commonly found in women, particularly those of the postmenopausal age range. While still relatively unknown how it's acquired or what causes it, doctors note that LS is not contagious.

The skin that is affected by LS becomes patchy white, shiny, and wrinkled, similar to how a parchment looks. This becomes prone to tearing and bleeding and may eventually lead to scarring. When left untreated, the scarring of LS may lead to problems in urinating, defecating, and sexual intercourse.

Albeit the genital mucosa is released, lacerations at the mucocutaneous junction can prompt introital narrowing. The orifice contribution is normal (leading to an 'hourglass' or 'figure of eight' circulation of infection). Different discoveries incorporate mutilation of the vulvar architecture, portrayed frequently by labial fusion, phimosis, and fissures of the clitoral hood.

How Normal Is Lichen Sclerosus?
Lichen sclerosus is uncommon. Approximately 200,000 individuals in the US have the condition. It influences individuals of all sexes. Girls, as well as women, are bound to foster the condition more than men.

LS is most widespread in females who have experienced menopause. It's almost certain to foster between ages 40 & 60. Girls who haven't begun adolescence likewise have a higher danger. Less ordinarily, lichen sclerosus influences guys who haven't been circumcised. The etiology remains obscure, even though proof focuses on a hereditary and, additionally, autoimmune disorder.

For instance, in an enormous observational cohort investigation of more than 1,000 ladies with lichen sclerosus, about 12% had a positive family background of LS. Backing for the latter hypothesis originates from the continuous relationship of other autoimmune issues like vitiligo, alopecia, thyrotoxicosis, pernicious anemia, and hypothyroidism in patients with lichen sclerosus.

As a result of the persistent tingling & scratching found in females with lichen sclerosus, this population is at an increased danger of vulvar carcinoma. Although patients most usually report pruritus, different side effects such as burning, irritation, tearing, and dyspareunia are found most of the time.

Since LS can be asymptomatic, the genuine commonness of the illness stays obscure. Commonness gauges range from 1:60 to around 1:1,000 *(AAFP, 2021)*.

How Does It Affect Females?
Lichen sclerosus in females is an ongoing inflammatory dermatitis, with an inclination for the anogenital part, which now and again can turn out to be extremely distorted (atrophy of the phimosis, labia minora, introital stenosis, and so on).

The majority of cases are analyzed in postmenopausal ladies, yet it can be seen in ladies of all ages. Lichen sclerosus is normally an extremely itchy condition, even though it can similarly be asymptomatic. It is related to an expanded danger of vulvar malignancy, even if it's not a premalignant condition itself.

It's also believed that LS may be considered a symptom of a more malignant condition called vulvar intraepithelial neoplasia (VIN). However, this still needs further analysis, which is usually done through a biopsy to get a proper diagnosis.

LS SYMPTOMS, CAUSES, AND CURES

People with mild lichen sclerosus may have no indications or signs before having them. The signs & symptoms generally influence the skin of the genital along with anal parts, yet may equally influence the skin of the upper body, upper arms, and bosoms.

They may cause the following:
• Uneasiness or agony
• Tearing or bleeding
• Redness
• Unpleasant sex
• Smooth white spots on your skin
• Wrinkled, blotchy patches
• Tingling (pruritus), which can be acute
• In critical cases, blistering, bleeding, or ulcerated lesions

Causes and Risk Factors
The origin for LS isn't clear; doctors speculate that various variables might be included, such as the following:

• Heredity
Lichen sclerosus is, by all accounts, more prevalent in certain families. Individuals who are hereditarily inclined to LS may

foster manifestations after encountering injury, trauma, or sexual maltreatment.

- Hyperactivity of the Immune System

LS in females might be an autoimmune syndrome, in which the body's immune system erroneously assaults and harms the skin. Ladies with lichen sclerosus are in more danger of mounting various other autoimmune disorders, like a few kinds of thyroid infection, diabetes, anemia, and alopecia areata, accompanied by vitiligo.

- Hormones

LS is more widespread in prepubescent & postmenopausal females, proposing that hormonal changes impact the illness. Notwithstanding, cures, for example, hormone replacement treatment or the use of progesterone or testosterone have not been demonstrated to be effective for females with LS.

- Urine

There is proof that urine may add to genital LS in males, in that urine drops may pool between the glans penis along with the prepuce, adding to lichen sclerosus in uncircumcised men. Nonetheless, whether pee has an impact on genital LS in females is not clear *(Women's, 2021)*.

Complications on LS may result in problems in urinating, sexual intercourse unpleasant sex, constipation, and a failure to withdraw the prepuce. People with LS are additionally at a greater risk of squamous cell carcinoma in the area concerned.

When to Visit a Doctor

Visit your physician when you see or experience the symptoms of LS described in this guide to get an expert's opinion. If you've previously been detected to have LS, see your physician every 6 to 12 months to be checked for any sort of skin changes or treatment adverse effects.

There are several things you can do to keep your skin from getting irritated or harmed. Do the following:

- Rinse with emollient soap rather than ordinary soap. Consult with your doctor or a pharmacist for suitable products
- Consistently apply a barrier ointment or cream, such as petroleum jelly, to affected areas.
- Wear silk or cotton underwear.
- Gently dab your genitals dry soon after peeing.
- Use vaginal lubricant in case having sex is painful.

Don't:
- Rub or scratch the affected skin.
- Wear restrictive or tight garments.
- Wash your underwear with strong detergent—simply use water

How Is Lichen Sclerosus Cured?
Unfortunately, at the moment, there is no treatment for lichen sclerosus. There are, however, ways to manage it.

Cortisone ointment applied to the vulva can give help and prevent lichen sclerosus from worsening. This is an enduring treatment and should be applied consistently—like once or twice a week, depending on what's recommended by your doctor.

When LS doesn't respond to topical treatments, surgery may be performed, especially to get rid of malignant symptoms. Also, surgery to get rid of the scarring in the outer layer of the vagina may be performed. This will greatly help those who are having problems with penetrative sex.

Frequent visits to the physician will be required, keeping tabs on the development or changes in areas affected by LS.

While there is no cure yet to completely get rid of LS, it's not a life-threatening condition. It's also not infectious. As long as it's treated well, symptoms may lessen and become more bearable.

One has the choice to help plan their care. Talk about treatment choices with your doctor to help you understand what type of treatment is best for you.

MANAGING LS THROUGH DIET AND LIFESTYLE

At the moment, managing LS through diet still requires more controlled studies. There are varied studies regarding the effectiveness of different LS-focused diets, however, if applicable to your condition, there's nothing wrong if you decide to give it a try.

One of the more well-known diet plans to manage lichen sclerosus is the low-oxalate diet. It's believed to affect the pain level of LS. This is also proven effective for some women, especially those with high levels of oxalate in their urine.

More about Low-oxalate Food
Here is a list of foods that are considered low-oxalate:
- Fish
- Meat
- Poultry
- Avocados
- Apples, peeled
- Melon
- Peaches*
- Plums*

- Grapes*
- Broccoli*
- Asparagus*
- Cauliflower
- Lettuce*
- Green peas
- Coffee*
- White chocolate
- Lightly steeped, mild green tea
- Dairy
- Vegetable oils
- Herbs & seasonings (white pepper, salt, basil, and cilantro)
- Beer*

*Food items fall under medium oxalate list, so consume in moderation.

Food to Avoid

On the other hand, here is a list of some of the foods you should avoid during the low-oxalate diet:
- Rhubarb
- Bran flakes
- Almonds
- Rice bran
- Beets
- Turnip greens
- Soy flour
- Buckwheat groats
- Boxed cereals
- Dried fruits
- Spinach, raw & cooked
- Nut
- Peanut butter
- Brown rice*
- Cocoa powder and hot chocolate
- Potatoes and sweet potatoes (including raw and other variants, such as French fries, baked, and potato chips)

*Falls under medium oxalate list.

Organic and Alternative Remedies for Lichen Sclerosus
There are alternative options that you can try alongside the usual treatment you're getting for your LS. Before trying them out, consult first with your doctor to ensure that you're getting the benefits of these alternative remedies and not making the condition worse. First of these remedies are herbs:

● Calendula
This is one of the herbs to have for skin disorders. It's antifungal, antibacterial, and antiseptic. Its injury-mending properties help fight contamination.

● Comfrey
Comfrey is used for its tissue recuperating benefits. Also called knit bone, it assists with combining back the harmed cells. Comfrey helps mend wounds in a brief time frame.

When used, make sure that the injured area is clean to allow the comfrey to work quickly and avoid contamination.

● Witch Hazel
It is an astringent and will aid in slightly drying the skin, without it over-drying. It also protects the skin from getting infections.

● Red Clover
It is utilized as an anti-inflammatory. It mends wounds and has certain phytoestrogen impacts. This has been known to help recuperate lichen in menopausal ladies.

● Plantain
It's a great herb to help ease the tingle on the skin. Its chemical herbal characteristics prevent the itch of lichen whenever used consistently.

These herbs are present in the only natural product specifically made to treat LS, Lisepten™.

Various Home Remedies

A few people don't react well to corticosteroids, even getting adverse reactions. For this situation, home remedies might be a safer option instead of creams and ointments. Some of these natural products may include the following:

1. Lavender essential oil – will help stop burning and itching.
2. Aloe vera gel – soothes skin and will help reduce inflammation. Apply a few times each day.
3. Baking soda – helps with inflammation. Add a tablespoon of this in water for soaking.
4. Coconut oil – alleviates tingling and burning.
5. Emu oil – an anti-inflammatory that eases irritation and swelling.
6. Magnesium – oral supplement used for lack of magnesium.
7. Borax – mixed with baking soda in hot water, will help with the inflammation.
8. Apple cider vinegar – soothes the infected skin, and can be applied to injuries with a cotton ball a couple of times each day
9. Castor oil – may help soothe skin. Mix 3 to 4 tbsp. of castor oil with a few drops of lavender oil, and store in a container. When the mixture becomes pasty, apply to sores daily.
10. Dietary modifications – Candida diet and probiotics may aid in soothing the LS symptoms since it wipes out yeast contamination which can be linked to LS.

Is There a Way to Prevent Getting Lichen Sclerosus?
Sadly, no. However, you may find ways to alleviate its symptoms by changing your lifestyle, some of which are, for example, to help decrease friction in the affected area that causes irritation. Try to:
• Stay away from long bicycle rides and horseback riding.
• Wear baggy underclothing and garments.
• Use unscented laundry detergent and soaps. Refrain from doing bubble baths. Bubbles can trigger irritation that exacerbates the tingling sensation in the affected areas.
• Change out of wet bathing suits and garments immediately.

There isn't a definite or specific lichen sclerosus diet plan. In any case, a few findings show that dietary changes can help ease the symptoms of LS, which for most is worth a shot.

THE LICHEN SCLEROSUS DIET

Like any other autoimmune condition, it's always necessary to assume that what you consume may affect or benefit your condition. In the previous chapter, different types of foods to avoid and consume have already been listed. You may start from there. Consulting with your doctor will also be beneficial as they may help you tailor the diet meal according to your needs.

Some researchers proposed that a low-oxalate diet can help lessen the symptoms of LS, but some counter-researches refute that claim. Thus, it's important to remember that this diet plan may or may not work for you. On the other hand, trying out the low-oxalate diet may still be beneficial, as there are studies that show how a usual diet, particularly in the west where consumed foods are usually processed and are high in salt, can aggravate its symptoms.

LS Diet Plan: Step-by-Step
Here is a planning guide you can follow to help you gently break into your LS diet journey.

<u>Curating your pantry</u>
For starters, it's expected that you'd want to properly tailor your pantry with the types of food that will become staples during this

diet plan and remove the ones that you need to stay away from. Here's a list of foods you need to stock up on the following:

- Vegetables, except for those which belong in the nightshade family
- Top-quality fish that are rich in omega-3 fatty acids
- Fermented foods, namely Sauerkraut, kombucha, kefir, kimchi, formed with water or coconut water
- Lean meats and liver
- Fruits, but not more than 2 to 3 a day to avoid overconsumption of fructose
- Vegetable oils, as well as avocado, olive, and coconut oils
- Meats such as beef, pork, chicken, turkey
- Some legumes like lentils, green peas, and black-eyed peas
- Dairy, particularly coconut milk

Collectively, this new eating regimen centers on consuming whole foods and those that don't include additives like sugar.

Now that you have an idea of what foods to stock up on, here are the types of food you need to refrain from consuming:

- Grains particularly bulgur wheat, corn grits, cornmeal, millet wheat, rice bran, and wheat berries (and except for corn bran, corn flour, flaxseed, hummus, oat bran, and white rice)
- Some legumes, nuts, and seeds, particularly pecans, garbanzos, and green beans
- Whole wheat products
- Nightshade vegetables like potatoes, peppers, tomatoes, and eggplants
- Soy milk and other soy products
- Fruits like grapefruit and kiwi

Exercise
Working out at your own speed is highly encouraged in this program. Exercise is great for women with lichen sclerosus as it can positively affect hormonal imbalance and may also revert your attention from the discomfort you're experiencing.

However, if experiencing a severe flare-up, do simple and easy exercises or take a break until it becomes bearable.

Some workouts you can try are strolling, sit-ups, running on a treadmill, and lifting weights to name a few. Biking, on the other hand, is not recommended because of the chafing, which may irritate the inflammation further. However, some use specialized bike seats and saddles that work for them. If you're able to acquire similar equipment, then go ahead and include biking in your workout regimen in moderation.

Additional tips when working out: make sure you also use a lubricant to lessen friction. Wear comfortable or loose apparel. Be cautious when swimming either in pools or the sea because the chemicals or saltwater may aggravate your condition.

A 7-DAY DIET PLAN

A sample of a 7-day diet plan for lichen sclerosus is shared below, but you can modify it according to your needs.

	Breakfast	Lunch	Snack	Dinner
Monday	Egg Roll Bowl	Asian Stir-Fry	Watermelon and Cucumber Drink	Beef and Live Burger
Tuesday	Cauliflower and Mushroom Bake	New York Steak and Steamed Broccoli	Grenade Salad	Chicken Broth
Wednesday	Buttered Eggs with Cheese	Bacon Chicken Bites	Zero Carb Pizza Crust	Creamy Low-FODMAP Fish Casserole
Thursday	Cauliflower and Mushroom Bake	Beef Heart	Healthy Broccoli with Cheese Sauce	Apricot-Glazed Salmon
Friday	Poached Eggs on a Toast	Crispy Pork Chop with Flavorful Brussels Sprouts	Plantain Strips	Roasted Broccoli and Salmon
Saturday	Cauliflower and Mushroom Bake	Chicken Broth	Pickle Fry	Bacon Chicken Bites
Sunday	Avocado Egg Toast	Apricot-Glazed Salmon	Green Coleslaw	Asian Stir-Fry

For week one, start with slowly transitioning from your regular diet to this new one. Slowly remove the food you need to stay away from and start stocking up on the food that won't worsen your symptoms. You can continue cooking your usual recipes but try to replace high-oxalate ingredients with better alternatives.

As you start this diet program, take notes of all the meals you prepared and how your body reacted. This way, you'll be able to track down which foods or ingredients may be beneficial or harmful to you.

You can also slowly transition into including light exercises to keep you active. Make sure that you're getting enough calories as you work out to avoid having problems later on.

In your second and third weeks, you're probably more used to your new lifestyle as well as how you prepare your meal plans for these weeks. Just continue what you have started, and if you have an appointment with a doctor during this period, make sure you share with your doctor the notes you took and what changes you've experienced so far. This way, your doctor will be able to advise you moving forward.

Egg Roll Bowl

Ingredients:
- 1 package of defrosted egg roll wrappers, cut into 0.5x3-inch per piece
- 1.5 lbs. ground pork
- 3 small cloves of garlic, minced
- 2 tsp. fresh ginger, peeled and minced
- 1/2 cup vegetable or chicken broth
- 1/3 cup coconut aminos
- 1.5 tsp. toasted sesame oil
- 1 9-oz. package pre-shredded cabbage
- 3-4 green onions, chopped
- sriracha sauce

Instructions:
1. Preheat the oven to 400°F.
2. Place wrappers on a baking sheet. Brush with a little olive oil.
3. Bake for about 5 minutes, or until golden brown.
4. In a large pan, heat 1 tbsp. of oil over medium-high heat.
5. Add raw meat. Cook for about 4-5 minutes, or until golden brown.
6. Drain or pat with a paper towel after removing from the pan.
7. Raw meat is browned in a pan
8. In the same pan, turn the heat to medium. Add garlic and ginger, and stir occasionally for about a minute.
9. Add cabbage slaw mix and most of the green onions. Cook for around 3 minutes until softened.
10. Add broth, coconut amino, and sesame oil. Stir well.
11. Scoop up the ingredients into a bowl.
12. Top with toasted egg roll wrappers, sriracha, and leftover green onions.

Green Coleslaw

Ingredients:
- 1/2 cup white distilled vinegar
- 1/4 cup granulated white sugar
- 1 tsp. kosher salt
- 1/4 tsp. black pepper
- 1/2 head green cabbage shredded

Instructions:
1. Stir together vinegar, sugar, salt, and pepper until well-combined and sugar is dissolved.
2. Place cabbage in a large bowl and pour vinegar mixture over it.
3. Stir to combine.
4. Let coleslaw sit for at least 30 minutes at room temperature, to let the flavors meld.
5. Serve with pulled pork, BBQ chicken, fish tacos, or as a side for a grilled feast.

Pickle Fry

Ingredients:
- 30 dill pickles, absorb excess moisture with paper towels
- 1/2 cup all-purpose flour
- 2 medium eggs
- 2 tbsp. pickle juice
- 1/2 tsp. garlic powder
- 1/3 cup bread crumbs
- 1/2 cup panko bread crumbs
- cooking spray

Instructions:
1. Pour flour into a bowl.
2. In a separate bowl, add regular bread crumbs, panko bread crumbs, and garlic powder. Mix everything well.
3. In another bowl, put the eggs and pickle juice. Whisk them well.
4. Take a few pickles and put them in the flour mixture. Then, dip them in the egg mixture, and finally in the crumb mixture. Press the pickles to coat them well.
5. Place the pickles in a single layer in the air fryer basket. Lightly coat the top of the pickles with cooking spray.
6. Cook them for 5 minutes at 400°F. After 5 minutes, take them out and again spray some oil. Cook for another 5 minutes.
7. Serve them hot with your favorite sauce.

Crispy Pork Chop with Flavorful Brussels Sprouts

Ingredients:
- 8 oz. pork chop, bone-in and center-cut
- 6 oz. brussels sprouts
- 1/2 tsp. ground black pepper
- 1 tsp. olive oil
- 1 tsp. maple syrup
- 1 tsp. Dijon mustard
- cooking spray

Instructions:
1. In a bowl, put the pork chop and coat it lightly with cooking spray. Add half of the black pepper over it.
2. Take another bowl and add the oil along with maple syrup, dijon mustard, and remaining black pepper. Whisk them well.
3. In the mixture, add Brussels sprouts and toss it.
4. Place the marinated pork chop on one side of the air fryer basket. On the other side, place the coated sprouts.
5. Heat the air fryer to 400°F.
6. Place the basket and cook it until the pork turns golden brown.
7. After it turns golden, cook it for another 10 minutes to make it more tender.

*black pepper is substituted with white pepper

New York Steak and Steamed Broccoli

Ingredients:
- 6 oz. New York Strip Steak, excess fat removed
- 3 cups broccoli florets
- 1/2 tsp. garlic, minced
- 1/2 tsp. sea salt
- 1/8 tsp. ground white pepper*

Instructions:
1. Preheat the broiler and broiler pan.
2. Rub both sides of the steak with garlic, salt, and pepper.
3. Place the steak on the hot broiling pan.
4. Broil for 7 to 15 minutes or until desired doneness has been achieved.
5. Steam broccoli in the microwave or stovetop using a bowl of 2-inch deep water.
6. Sprinkle it with salt and pepper to taste.
7. Transfer steak onto a plate.
8. Transfer steamed broccoli to the side of the steak or in a separate bowl.
9. Serve immediately.

*black pepper is substituted with white pepper

Asian Stir-Fry

Ingredients:
- 1 lb. beef or chicken, sliced
- 1/2 tsp. garlic powder
- 3/4 tsp. ground ginger
- 2 lb. stir-fry vegetables, chopped
- 1/4 cup apple cider vinegar
- 1/2 tsp. sea salt
- 1/8 cup honey
- 1 cup broth
- 6 tbsp. coconut aminos

Instructions:
1. In a stock pot over high heat, put and mix all the ingredients.
2. Bring to a boil. Then, lower the heat down to medium.
3. Cover the pot and allow the mixture to simmer for 20 minutes, or until the meat has cooked through and the vegetables are sufficiently tender.
4. Serve while hot.

Bacon Chicken Bites

Ingredients:
- 1 large chicken breast, large, cut into 22 to 27 small pieces
- 8-9 thin bacon slices, chop each into 3
- 3 tbsp. garlic powder

Instructions:
1. Preheat the oven to 400°F.
2. Use aluminum foil to line a baking tray.
3. In a bowl, place the garlic powder. Dip each chicken piece into the garlic powder.
4. Wrap a bacon piece around a chicken piece. After wrapping, arrange the bacon-chicken pieces on the baking tray.
5. Bake until the bacon becomes crispy, for about 25 to 30 minutes. About 15 minutes into baking, turn the chicken pieces.
6. Remove from the oven and arrange on a serving plate.
7. Serve and enjoy.

Chicken Broth

Ingredients:
- 1 chicken carcass from a leftover roast chicken or bones
- 2 cloves of garlic
- water
- Optional: carrot or parsnip tops, leftover vegetable peelings, and herbs

Instructions:
1. Cover chicken bones with water, whether cooking in a large stockpot, a pressure cooker, or a slow cooker.
2. For the slow cooker, cook on high for 4 hours.
3. For the pressure cooker, set it to cook for an hour.
4. For the stockpot, set it on low simmer for 3 to 4 hours.
5. Once the time is up, strain the liquid from the broth through a sieve into a large bowl or container.
6. Discard the bones and garlic.
7. Keep the liquid, and pour it into a container.

Zero Carb Pizza Crust

Ingredients:
- 10 oz. canned chicken
- 1 oz. grated parmesan cheese
- 1 large egg

Instructions:
1. Drain the canned chicken thoroughly, getting as much moisture out as possible.
2. Spread chicken on a baking sheet lined with a silicone mat.
3. Bake at 350°F for 10 minutes to dry out the chicken.
4. Once it's done, remove it and place it in a mixing bowl. Increase the heat of the oven to 500°F.
5. Add cheese and egg to the bowl with chicken and mix.
6. Pour the mixture onto a baking sheet lined with a silicone mat.
7. Spread thinly. Place parchment paper on top and use a rolling pin to do so.
8. Optional: With a spatula, press in the edges of the crust to create a ridge, to keep any topping from falling off.
9. Bake the crust for 8-10 minutes at 500°F.
10. Remove the crust from the oven.
11. Add desired toppings and bake for another 6-10 minutes at 500°F. Toppings will dictate the final cook time.
12. Remove from the oven and allow to cool for a few minutes.
13. Serve and enjoy.

Buttered Eggs with Cheese

Ingredients:
- 2 eggs
- cheese

Instructions:
1. Boil a couple of eggs.
2. Once they're done, cut them in half.
3. Place them on a small plate.
4. Cut the cheese into medium-sized strips.
5. Layer the strips of cheese beside the boiled eggs.
6. Enjoy your breakfast.

Poached Eggs on a Toast

Ingredients:
- water in pan 1 1/2 inches deep
- 1 tsp. white vinegar
- 1 egg
- sea salt
- freshly cracked white pepper*
- 1 slice buttered toast

Instructions:
1. Fill up a pan with water up to 1-1/2 deep. Add vinegar.
2. Let it simmer over medium heat.
3. Crack open an egg into a bowl.
4. As the water simmers, use a slotted spoon and stir the mixture clockwise, creating a swirling motion.
5. Gently slide the egg into the water.
6. Cover the pan and turn off the heat.
7. Leave the eggs to poach until the whites are firm enough, or about 3 minutes and 45 seconds.
8. Take the egg with a slotted spoon to drain out the water.
9. Slide the egg into a buttered toast. Season with sea salt and pepper.
10. Serve immediately and enjoy.

*black pepper is substituted with white pepper

Avocado Egg Toast

Ingredients:
- 1/4 avocado
- 1/8 tsp. garlic powder
- 1/4 tsp. ground pepper
- 1 pc. fried egg
- 1 slice toasted whole-wheat bread
- optional: 1 tbsp. scallion
- optional: 1 tsp. sriracha

Instructions:
1. Mash the avocado together with the garlic powder and pepper in a bowl.
2. Put the mashed avocado on the toast.
3. Add the egg on top then garnish with scallion and sriracha.
4. Serve immediately.

*black pepper is substituted with white pepper and whole wheat bread is substituted with rye or white bread

Apricot-Glazed Salmon

Ingredients:
- 1-1/3 pounds wild salmon filets
- 1/4 tsp. of crushed white pepper*
- 1 tbsp. virgin olive oil
- 1/2 cup of sodium-free vegetable broth
- 1 tbsp. Dijon mustard
- 1/3 cup of 100% apricot fruit spread
- 1 tsp. minced garlic

Instructions:
1. Preheat the grill over medium heat.
2. Pat salmon dry with a paper towel and cut it into four slices.
3. Season the skinless side with black pepper.
4. Wrap each piece with aluminum foil, with the skin side down. Fold the foil around the salmon securely to prevent oil from leaking.
5. In a bowl, combine the remaining ingredients.
6. Pour the mixture over the salmon slices.
7. Grill salmon for ten minutes.
8. Once cooked, allow the grilled filet to cool down before unwrapping.
9. Plate nicely and garnish with your favorite herbs before serving.

*black pepper is substituted with white pepper

Roasted Broccoli and Salmon

Ingredients;
- 1-1/2 lbs. or 1 bunch broccoli, cut into florets
- 4 tbsp. avocado oil, divided
- 1 tsp salt
- 1 tsp pepper
- 4 pcs. salmon filets, deskinned
- 1 pc. jalapeño or red Fresno chile, deseeded and sliced into thin rings
- 2 tbsp. unseasoned rice vinegar
- 2 tbsp. capers, drained

Instructions:
Preheat the oven to 400° F.
2. Place broccoli florets on a large, rimmed baking sheet. Drizzle with 2 tbsp. avocado oil and season with salt and pepper.
3. Roast the florets in the oven for 12 or 15 minutes. Toss occasionally.
4. Remove from the oven when the florets are crisp-tender and browned.
5. Gently rub the salmon filets with 1 tbsp. of the avocado oil. Season with salt and pepper.
6. Place the salmon in the middle of the baking sheet. Move the florets to the sides of the baking sheet.
7. Roast the filet for 10 to 15 minutes or until the filets turn opaque throughout.
8. In a small bowl, combine the vinegar, chile rings, and a pinch of salt. Let the mixture sit for about 10 minutes, allowing the chile rings to soften a bit.
9. Add the capers and the remaining avocado oil. Add salt and pepper to taste.
10. Drizzle chile vinaigrette over the roasted broccoli and salmon just before serving.

Creamy Low-FODMAP Fish Casserole

Ingredients:
- 1-1/2 lb. white fish, serving-sized pieces
- 2 tbsp. olive oil
- 2 tbsp. small capers
- 1 lb. broccoli
- 1 oz. grass-fed butter
- 6 scallions
- 1 tbsp. Dijon mustard
- 1 tbsp. dried barley
- 1 tsp. salt
- 1/4 tsp. ground white pepper*

Instructions:
1. Set the oven temperature to 400°F.
2. Cut the broccoli into small florets with the stems included. Fry the broccoli for 3-5 minutes until soft and golden, then add salt and pepper.
3. Add the finely chopped scallions and the capers, then fry for another 2-3 minutes.
4. Grease the baking dish with butter and add in the fried vegetables.
5. Add the white fish to the vegetable mix.
6. In an oven-ready plate, mix the parsley, mustard, and whipping cream. Add the fish and vegetable mix and top with some butter.
7. Bake for 20-30 minutes or until fully cooked then serve.
8. In this particular recipe, broccoli is considered a high-FODMAP vegetable.

*black pepper is substituted with white pepper

Grenade Salad

Ingredients:
- 4 cups arugula
- 1 large avocado
- 1/2 cup sliced fennel
- 1/2 cup sliced Anjou pears
- 1/4 cup pomegranate seeds

Instructions:
1. Mix all the ingredients except for the pomegranate seeds.
2. After mixing well, add the seeds. Mix again.
3. Serve with any type of desired dressing.

Healthy Broccoli with Cheese Sauce

Ingredients:
- 6 cups broccoli florets
- 10 tbsp. milk
- 1.5 oz. Mexican cheese, crumbled
- 4 tsp. Aji Amarillo paste
- 6 pcs. saltine crackers
- cooking spray

Instructions:
1. Coat the broccoli florets lightly with cooking spray.
2. Place half of the florets in the air fryer basket and cook them for 8 minutes at 375°F.
3. Once cooked, repeat the process with the remaining florets.
4. In a blender, add milk, cheese, and Amarillo paste, along with saltines. Blend until the mixture becomes smooth.
5. Pour the sauce into a microwaveable bowl. Microwave the mixture for 30 seconds.
6. Serve the broccoli with the cheese sauce.

Watermelon and Cucumber Drink

Ingredients:
- 1 cup watermelon, deseeded
- 1/2 cup crushed ice
- 1/2 piece cucumber, peeled, deseeded
- 1/4 tsp. green stevia

Instructions:
1. Combine all ingredients in a blender. Process until smooth.
2. Serve immediately.

Plantain Strips

Ingredients:
- 2 pcs. overripe plantain, peeled and sliced into strips
- 1/2 tbsp. coconut oil

Instructions:
1. Pour oil into a non-stick pan set over medium heat.
2. Fry plantain strips in hot oil until golden brown but not crisp.
3. Remove strips from hot oil.
4. Place cooked plantains on a plate lined with a paper towel to drain excess grease.
5. Serve immediately.

Cauliflower and Mushroom Bake

Ingredients:
- 3 cups cauliflower florets
- 1 cup fresh mushroom, chopped
- 1/2 cup red onion, chopped
- 1/3 cup green onion, chopped
- 2 garlic cloves, finely chopped
- 2 tsp. apple cider vinegar
- 2 tsp. lemon juice
- 1/2 tsp. salt
- 1/4 tsp. white pepper
- 1 tbsp. olive oil

Instructions:
1. Preheat the oven to 350°F. Lightly grease a baking pan.
2. Combine red onion, cauliflower, olive oil, garlic, mushroom, apple cider vinegar, lemon juice, salt, and pepper in a bowl. Mix well.
3. Pour the mixture into the greased baking pan.
4. Place inside the oven and bake for 45 minutes. Stir.
5. When vegetables are golden brown and tender, remove them from the oven.
6. Garnish with green onions. Serve and enjoy.

*black pepper is substituted with white pepper

Beef and Liver Burger

Ingredients:
- 1-1/4 lb. ground beef
- 1/4 lb. chicken livers
- 1 tsp. sea salt
- 1/2 red onion, peeled
- 1 tsp. ground white pepper*
- 1-1/2 tsp. coriander
- 1 tsp. poultry seasoning

Instructions:
1. Put the liver and onion in a food processor. Pulse until mush.
2. Pour in the ground beef and the remaining spices. Pulse until the mixture is blended, or for roughly a minute.
3. Prepare a saucer with water to wet your hands before shaping the patties.
4. Shape 4-inch wide patties with the mixture.
5. Cook or grill the patties.
6. Serve in a hamburger bun or on a lettuce wrap.

*black pepper is substituted with white pepper

Beef Heart

Ingredients:
- 1 tbsp. ghee
- 4 slices beef heart, about an inch thick
- 2 tbsp. olive oil, rosemary-infused or plain
- salt
- white pepper*

Instructions:
1. Take heart slices from the marinade and pat dry.
2. Heat a cast-iron skillet with the ghee on a high flame for 2-3 minutes.
3. Lay the meat in the skillet. The temperature should be high enough to sizzle.
4. Cook for 5 minutes on each side until nicely browned on the outside but still pink in the middle.
5. Drizzle with rosemary-infused olive oil.
6. Serve with a salad of choice.

*black pepper is substituted with white pepper

CONCLUSION

Since it is still unknown how LS is acquired, the medical field is also in the dark as to how to prevent it from starting.

Several studies talk about its symptoms and how different food affects it, whether to ease the symptoms or worsen them. Getting diagnosed as early as possible will help in curbing the symptoms from worsening.

Experts advise women to openly discuss with their gynecologists if they notice skin lesions or changes around their private area, or experience tingling or itchiness. A change in attitude regarding this condition will greatly benefit you.

Thank you again for getting this guide.

If you found this guide helpful, please take the time to share your thoughts and post a review. It'd be greatly appreciated!

References

All about lichen sclerosus: Symptoms, causes, and treatment. (2022, January 21). Healthline. https://www.healthline.com/health/lichen-sclerosus.

Beginner's guide to the low-oxalate diet | theralogix balanced living blog. (2021, July 20). Balanced Living Blog. https://blog.theralogix.com/low-oxalate-diet/.

CSG, M. B. M., RD, CSR. (2021, May 18). Top 10 low oxalate beans. The Kidney Dietitian. https://www.thekidneydietitian.org/low-oxalate-beans/.

Dietary changes to prevent calcium oxalate stones. (n.d.). Retrieved September 1, 2022, from https://mydoctor.kaiserpermanente.org/ncal/Images/Dietary%20Changes%20to%20Prevent%20Calcium%20Oxalate%20Stones_tcm75-194243.pdf.

Diseasemaps. (n.d.). Is it advisable to do exercise when affected by lichen sclerosus? which activities would you suggest and how intense should they be? Diseasemaps. Retrieved September 1, 2022, from https://www.diseasemaps.org/lichen-sclerosus/top-questions/exercice-and-sports/.

Fugo, J., & *, N. (2020, December 12). 040: Lichen sclerosus help with diet and physical therapy W/ dr. Jessica Drummond. Skinterrupt. Retrieved September 1, 2022, from https://www.skinterrupt.com/lichen-sclerosus-diet-physical-therapy/.

Hospital, T. R. W. (n.d.). Lichen sclerosus. The Royal Women's Hospital. Retrieved September 1, 2022, from https://www.thewomens.org.au/health-information/vulva-vagina/vulva-vagina-problems/lichen-sclerosus.

How to eat a low oxalate diet | kidney stone evaluation and treatment program. (n.d.). Retrieved September 1, 2022, from https://kidneystones.uchicago.edu/how-to-eat-a-low-oxalate-

diet/#:~:text=PASTA%20RICE%20AND
%20GRAINS&text=Millet%20and%20bulger%2C%20wheat
%20berries,bran%20are%20popular%20and%20safe

Low oxalate diet - what you need to know. Drugs.com. (n.d.). Retrieved September 1, 2022, from https://www.drugs.com/cg/low-oxalate-diet.html.

Low oxalate diet » arizona digestive health. (n.d.). Retrieved September 1, 2022, from https://www.arizonadigestivehealth.com/low-oxalate-diet/

Marfatia, Y., Surani, A., & Baxi, R. (2019). Genital lichen sclerosus et atrophicus in females: An update. Indian Journal of Sexually Transmitted Diseases and AIDS, 40(1), 6–12. https://doi.org/10.4103/ijstd.IJSTD_23_19.

Mazeski, M. (2022, August 3). Stem cell therapy Chicago: Regenerative Medicine & Stem Cells Specialist. Stem Cell Chicago. Retrieved September 1, 2022, from https://stemcelldr.com/lichen-sclerosus-cure.

McNulty, R. (2020, September 9). The 7-day diet detox plan. Muscle & Fitness. https://www.muscleandfitness.com/muscle-fitness-hers/hers-nutrition/7-day-meal-plan-clean-your-diet/.

myDr. (2017, May 23). Lichen sclerosus. MyDr.Com.Au. https://www.mydr.com.au/womens-health/lichen-sclerosus/.

Skin support. Home | Skin Support. (n.d.). Retrieved September 1, 2022, from http://www.skinsupport.org.uk/conditions-details/lichen-sclerosus-females.

Staff, F. E. (2022, August 8). Lichen sclerosus. familydoctor.org. Retrieved September 1, 2022, from https://familydoctor.org/condition/lichen-sclerosus/.

The beginner's guide to autoimmune protocol diet | ultimate paleo guide. (n.d.). Https://Ultimatepaleoguide.Com/. Retrieved September 1, 2022, from https://ultimatepaleoguide.com/

autoimmune-protocol/.

What you should know about lichen sclerosus | lichen sclerosus causes. (n.d.). Thinx | Thinx Teens | Speax. Retrieved September 1, 2022, from https://www.thinx.com/speax/blogs/foreword/lichen-sclerosus-signs-symptoms-treatment.

Made in the USA
Monee, IL
03 February 2023

26923100R00028